DIY Sunscreen

30 Perfect Organic Sunscreen Recipes With Essential Oils

Table of content

Introduction

Summertime is the time for fun.

It's time to get out in the sun and soak up some rays, it's time to head out to the beach and have fun in the sand, and it's time to indulge in all of the summertime activities that this time of year brings, but you need to do it the right way.

If you have your skin exposed without any kind of protection, you are just asking for problems. Dry skin, peeling skin, sun burns, and callouses all form, not to mention the other, smaller issues that can crop up as well, including sun spots, wrinkles, or other signs of being out in the weather.

Of course the only way to avoid any of these problems is to stay indoors out of the rays, or to wear winter style clothing that will cover you from head to toe, but you know that's not at all practical, especially if you want to get out and have fun in some of the summertime activities.

So what do you do?

"I spend so much time trying to stick with the organics and healthy choices."

"I do my best to avoid chemicals and other things I can't pronounce."

"I want to do things the natural way, and avoid any harsh chemicals."

These are just a few of the reasons many choose to use organic sun lotion, but there are many, many more. You know if you want to do this absolutely your way, you are going to have to make it yourself. And that is where this book comes in.

In it you are going to find the recipes you need to make your very own sun tan lotion, and know for certain that there is nothing inside that you don't want to put on your skin. To make it even better, you are going to be able to choose other benefits that come from the use of essential oils in your lotions.

Once you try your own lotion even once, you are going to be hooked, and you won't ever want to change your routine again. This book is going to show you just what you need to turn your idea into a reality, and in no time at all you are going to have your very own lotion, specific to your own needs.

So what are you waiting for? The sun isn't waiting for anyone, and neither should you!

Chapter 1 – Getting Started

When it comes to the essential oils and the sunscreen you wish to make, the possibilities are endless. So, for starters, I have included the recipe you will need for the base of the sunscreen.

This is going to give you all the protection you need, plus moisture where you need it the most. You can add the essential oils as you please until you get the scent you love!

Remember to purchase only organics for all of these ingredients. You can find them in a variety of local stores, or order them online. Amazon has everything you need and then some.

The Base Lotion Recipe

¾ cup coconut oil

½ cup shea butter

¼ cup mango butter

1/3 cup bees wax

Almond oil

1 ½ tablespoon zinc oxide

To make this base, all you need to do is warm all the ingredients on the stove. You don't want them to be so hot that they burn you, but warm enough that they can be mixed with a blender and easily combined.

Add the almond oil last, and add it to your preferred consistency. Your lotion isn't going to harden much, so work until you are happy with it, then add in the oils.

Easiest Ever Sunscreen

5 drops rose oil

5 drops orange

3 drops lemongrass

Base

Directions:

In a mixing bowl, blend all of the ingredients, first the base for the sunscreen, the zinc oxide, and the oils. You can follow the exact measurements that I have suggested for the oils, or you can add or take away as many drops as you like.

You are going to get incredible benefits from all the oils regardless of how much you use, but you will get more benefits depending on how much you use.

Use your blender until the mix is light and whipped, then transfer to a glass jar.

Store with the lid screwed on tightly, and massage into your skin when you are ready to use.

The Sun Shield

10 drops lemon oil

5 drops orange oil

5 drops wild orange

Base

Directions:

In a mixing bowl, blend all of the ingredients, first the base for the sunscreen, the zinc oxide, and the oils. You can follow the exact measurements that I have suggested for the oils, or you can add or take away as many drops as you like.

You are going to get incredible benefits from all the oils regardless of how much you use, but you will get more benefits depending on how much you use.

Use your blender until the mix is light and whipped, then transfer to a glass jar.

Store with the lid screwed on tightly, and massage into your skin when you are ready to use.

The Field Day Winner

10 drops lavender

5 drops orange

5 drops patchouli

Base

Directions:

In a mixing bowl, blend all of the ingredients, first the base for the sunscreen, the zinc oxide, and the oils. You can follow the exact measurements that I have suggested for the oils, or you can add or take away as many drops as you like.

You are going to get incredible benefits from all the oils regardless of how much you use, but you will get more benefits depending on how much you use.

Use your blender until the mix is light and whipped, then transfer to a glass jar.

Store with the lid screwed on tightly, and massage into your skin when you are ready to use.

Mom's Favorite Sunscreen

10 drops peppermint

5 drops spearmint

7 drops rose

Base

Directions:

In a mixing bowl, blend all of the ingredients, first the base for the sunscreen, the zinc oxide, and the oils. You can follow the exact measurements that I have suggested for the oils, or you can add or take away as many drops as you like.

You are going to get incredible benefits from all the oils regardless of how much you use, but you will get more benefits depending on how much you use.

Use your blender until the mix is light and whipped, then transfer to a glass jar.

Store with the lid screwed on tightly, and massage into your skin when you are ready to use.

Fun Time In The Sun Time

8 drops tea tree

8 drops peppermint

9 drops lemon

Base

Directions:

In a mixing bowl, blend all of the ingredients, first the base for the sunscreen, the zinc oxide, and the oils. You can follow the exact measurements that I have suggested for the oils, or you can add or take away as many drops as you like.

You are going to get incredible benefits from all the oils regardless of how much you use, but you will get more benefits depending on how much you use.

Use your blender until the mix is light and whipped, then transfer to a glass jar.

Store with the lid screwed on tightly, and massage into your skin when you are ready to use.

Wildflower Blossom

10 drops lavender

10 drops lilac

5 drops geranium

Base

Directions:

In a mixing bowl, blend all of the ingredients, first the base for the sunscreen, the zinc oxide, and the oils. You can follow the exact measurements that I have suggested for the oils, or you can add or take away as many drops as you like.

You are going to get incredible benefits from all the oils regardless of how much you use, but you will get more benefits depending on how much you use.

Use your blender until the mix is light and whipped, then transfer to a glass jar.

Store with the lid screwed on tightly, and massage into your skin when you are ready to use.

Chapter 2 – Any Time Sunscreens

The Picnic Basket

10 drops chamomile

5 drops lemongrass

3 drops apple essential oil

Base

Directions:

In a mixing bowl, blend all of the ingredients, first the base for the sunscreen, the zinc oxide, and the oils. You can follow the exact measurements that I have suggested for the oils, or you can add or take away as many drops as you like.

You are going to get incredible benefits from all the oils regardless of how much you use, but you will get more benefits depending on how much you use.

Use your blender until the mix is light and whipped, then transfer to a glass jar.

Store with the lid screwed on tightly, and massage into your skin when you are ready to use.

The Fisherman's Friend

10 drops tea tree

5 drops patchouli

5 drops garlic

Base

Directions:

In a mixing bowl, blend all of the ingredients, first the base for the sunscreen, the zinc oxide, and the oils. You can follow the exact measurements that I have suggested for the oils, or you can add or take away as many drops as you like.

You are going to get incredible benefits from all the oils regardless of how much you use, but you will get more benefits depending on how much you use.

Use your blender until the mix is light and whipped, then transfer to a glass jar.

Store with the lid screwed on tightly, and massage into your skin when you are ready to use.

The Tan Lines

8 drops chrysanthemum

8 drops rose

5 drops geranium

Base

Directions:

In a mixing bowl, blend all of the ingredients, first the base for the sunscreen, the zinc oxide, and the oils. You can follow the exact measurements that I have suggested for the oils, or you can add or take away as many drops as you like.

You are going to get incredible benefits from all the oils regardless of how much you use, but you will get more benefits depending on how much you use.

Use your blender until the mix is light and whipped, then transfer to a glass jar.

Store with the lid screwed on tightly, and massage into your skin when you are ready to use.

The Beach Day Delight

15 drops lemon

5 drops lemongrass

Base

Directions:

In a mixing bowl, blend all of the ingredients, first the base for the sunscreen, the zinc oxide, and the oils. You can follow the exact measurements that I have suggested for the oils, or you can add or take away as many drops as you like.

You are going to get incredible benefits from all the oils regardless of how much you use, but you will get more benefits depending on how much you use.

Use your blender until the mix is light and whipped, then transfer to a glass jar.

Store with the lid screwed on tightly, and massage into your skin when you are ready to use.

The Sunsets and Roses

10 drops rose

8 drops sandalwood

8 drops orange

8 drops wild orange

Base

Directions:

In a mixing bowl, blend all of the ingredients, first the base for the sunscreen, the zinc oxide, and the oils. You can follow the exact measurements that I have suggested for the oils, or you can add or take away as many drops as you like.

You are going to get incredible benefits from all the oils regardless of how much you use, but you will get more benefits depending on how much you use.

Use your blender until the mix is light and whipped, then transfer to a glass jar.

Store with the lid screwed on tightly, and massage into your skin when you are ready to use.

The Crazy Days

10 drops sandalwood

5 drops lavender

5 drops lilac

Base

Directions:

In a mixing bowl, blend all of the ingredients, first the base for the sunscreen, the zinc oxide, and the oils. You can follow the exact measurements that I have suggested for the oils, or you can add or take away as many drops as you like.

You are going to get incredible benefits from all the oils regardless of how much you use, but you will get more benefits depending on how much you use.

Use your blender until the mix is light and whipped, then transfer to a glass jar.

Store with the lid screwed on tightly, and massage into your skin when you are ready to use.

Chapter 3 – Bonus Blends Sunscreen

The Acne Buster

15 drops tea tree

5 drops myrrh

5 drops lemongrass

Base

Directions:

In a mixing bowl, blend all of the ingredients, first the base for the sunscreen, the zinc oxide, and the oils. You can follow the exact measurements that I have suggested for the oils, or you can add or take away as many drops as you like.

You are going to get incredible benefits from all the oils regardless of how much you use, but you will get more benefits depending on how much you use.

Use your blender until the mix is light and whipped, then transfer to a glass jar.

Store with the lid screwed on tightly, and massage into your skin when you are ready to use.

The Wrinkle Eraser

10 drops myrrh

10 drops chamomile

5 drops lemon

Base

Directions:

In a mixing bowl, blend all of the ingredients, first the base for the sunscreen, the zinc oxide, and the oils. You can follow the exact measurements that I have suggested for the oils, or you can add or take away as many drops as you like.

You are going to get incredible benefits from all the oils regardless of how much you use, but you will get more benefits depending on how much you use.

Use your blender until the mix is light and whipped, then transfer to a glass jar.

Store with the lid screwed on tightly, and massage into your skin when you are ready to use.

The Spotifyer

10 drops lemon

10 drops peppermint

6 drops orange

5 drops tea tree

Base

Directions:

In a mixing bowl, blend all of the ingredients, first the base for the sunscreen, the zinc oxide, and the oils. You can follow the exact measurements that I have suggested for the oils, or you can add or take away as many drops as you like.

You are going to get incredible benefits from all the oils regardless of how much you use, but you will get more benefits depending on how much you use.

Use your blender until the mix is light and whipped, then transfer to a glass jar.

Store with the lid screwed on tightly, and massage into your skin when you are ready to use.

The Fair Skinned Delight

10 drops cinnamon

10 drops peppermint

Base

Directions:

In a mixing bowl, blend all of the ingredients, first the base for the sunscreen, the zinc oxide, and the oils. You can follow the exact measurements that I have suggested for the oils, or you can add or take away as many drops as you like.

You are going to get incredible benefits from all the oils regardless of how much you use, but you will get more benefits depending on how much you use.

Use your blender until the mix is light and whipped, then transfer to a glass jar.

Store with the lid screwed on tightly, and massage into your skin when you are ready to use.

The Princess and the Pauper

10 drops chamomile

5 drops basil

5 drops ginger

Base

Directions:

In a mixing bowl, blend all of the ingredients, first the base for the sunscreen, the zinc oxide, and the oils. You can follow the exact measurements that I have suggested for the oils, or you can add or take away as many drops as you like.

You are going to get incredible benefits from all the oils regardless of how much you use, but you will get more benefits depending on how much you use.

Use your blender until the mix is light and whipped, then transfer to a glass jar.

Store with the lid screwed on tightly, and massage into your skin when you are ready to use.

The Glow

10 drops goldenseal

10 drops myrrh

10 drops frankincense

Base

Directions:

In a mixing bowl, blend all of the ingredients, first the base for the sunscreen, the zinc oxide, and the oils. You can follow the exact measurements that I have suggested for the oils, or you can add or take away as many drops as you like.

You are going to get incredible benefits from all the oils regardless of how much you use, but you will get more benefits depending on how much you use.

Use your blender until the mix is light and whipped, then transfer to a glass jar.

Store with the lid screwed on tightly, and massage into your skin when you are ready to use.

Chapter 4 – Scents and Senses Sunscreens

The Rosewood Bliss

10 drops rose

6 drops cedar wood

5 drops frankincense

Base

Directions:

In a mixing bowl, blend all of the ingredients, first the base for the sunscreen, the zinc oxide, and the oils. You can follow the exact measurements that I have suggested for the oils, or you can add or take away as many drops as you like.

You are going to get incredible benefits from all the oils regardless of how much you use, but you will get more benefits depending on how much you use.

Use your blender until the mix is light and whipped, then transfer to a glass jar.

Store with the lid screwed on tightly, and massage into your skin when you are ready to use.

Lilacs and Lilies

5 drops lavender

5 drops lilac

5 drops pine

3 drops lemongrass

Base

Directions:

In a mixing bowl, blend all of the ingredients, first the base for the sunscreen, the zinc oxide, and the oils. You can follow the exact measurements that I have suggested for the oils, or you can add or take away as many drops as you like.

You are going to get incredible benefits from all the oils regardless of how much you use, but you will get more benefits depending on how much you use.

Use your blender until the mix is light and whipped, then transfer to a glass jar.

Store with the lid screwed on tightly, and massage into your skin when you are ready to use.

Sunny Grass

10 drops anise

5 drops cardamom

5 drops cinnamon

4 drops lemongrass

Base

Directions:

In a mixing bowl, blend all of the ingredients, first the base for the sunscreen, the zinc oxide, and the oils. You can follow the exact measurements that I have suggested for the oils, or you can add or take away as many drops as you like.

You are going to get incredible benefits from all the oils regardless of how much you use, but you will get more benefits depending on how much you use.

Use your blender until the mix is light and whipped, then transfer to a glass jar.

Store with the lid screwed on tightly, and massage into your skin when you are ready to use.

Mountain Meadow

10 drops pine

5 drops cedar wood

5 drops tea tree

Base

Directions:

In a mixing bowl, blend all of the ingredients, first the base for the sunscreen, the zinc oxide, and the oils. You can follow the exact measurements that I have suggested for the oils, or you can add or take away as many drops as you like.

You are going to get incredible benefits from all the oils regardless of how much you use, but you will get more benefits depending on how much you use.

Use your blender until the mix is light and whipped, then transfer to a glass jar.

Store with the lid screwed on tightly, and massage into your skin when you are ready to use.

Sunflowers and Poppies

10 drops clary sage

5 drops eucalyptus

4 drops mint

Base

Directions:

In a mixing bowl, blend all of the ingredients, first the base for the sunscreen, the zinc oxide, and the oils. You can follow the exact measurements that I have suggested for the oils, or you can add or take away as many drops as you like.

You are going to get incredible benefits from all the oils regardless of how much you use, but you will get more benefits depending on how much you use.

Use your blender until the mix is light and whipped, then transfer to a glass jar.

Store with the lid screwed on tightly, and massage into your skin when you are ready to use.

The Birds and the Bees

10 drops rose

10 drops lavender

5 drops eucalyptus

5 drops spearmint

Base

Directions:

In a mixing bowl, blend all of the ingredients, first the base for the sunscreen, the zinc oxide, and the oils. You can follow the exact measurements that I have suggested for the oils, or you can add or take away as many drops as you like.

You are going to get incredible benefits from all the oils regardless of how much you use, but you will get more benefits depending on how much you use.

Use your blender until the mix is light and whipped, then transfer to a glass jar.

Store with the lid screwed on tightly, and massage into your skin when you are ready to use.

Chapter 5 – All the Best of All the Rest

The Life is Good Blend

6 drops peppermint

6 drops spearmint

5 drops eucalyptus

Base

Directions:

In a mixing bowl, blend all of the ingredients, first the base for the sunscreen, the zinc oxide, and the oils. You can follow the exact measurements that I have suggested for the oils, or you can add or take away as many drops as you like.

You are going to get incredible benefits from all the oils regardless of how much you use, but you will get more benefits depending on how much you use.

Use your blender until the mix is light and whipped, then transfer to a glass jar.

Store with the lid screwed on tightly, and massage into your skin when you are ready to use.

The Wandering Gypsy

10 drops patchouli

5 drops fir

5 drops grapefruit

Base

Directions:

In a mixing bowl, blend all of the ingredients, first the base for the sunscreen, the zinc oxide, and the oils. You can follow the exact measurements that I have suggested for the oils, or you can add or take away as many drops as you like.

You are going to get incredible benefits from all the oils regardless of how much you use, but you will get more benefits depending on how much you use.

Use your blender until the mix is light and whipped, then transfer to a glass jar.

Store with the lid screwed on tightly, and massage into your skin when you are ready to use.

The Happy Hippy Hippy Hooray

10 drops basil

6 drops tea tree

6 drops frankincense

Base

Directions:

In a mixing bowl, blend all of the ingredients, first the base for the sunscreen, the zinc oxide, and the oils. You can follow the exact measurements that I have suggested for the oils, or you can add or take away as many drops as you like.

You are going to get incredible benefits from all the oils regardless of how much you use, but you will get more benefits depending on how much you use.

Use your blender until the mix is light and whipped, then transfer to a glass jar.

Store with the lid screwed on tightly, and massage into your skin when you are ready to use.

The Wanderlust

10 drops pine

10 drops fir

5 drops grapefruit

5 drops orange

5 drops lemongrass

Base

Directions:

In a mixing bowl, blend all of the ingredients, first the base for the sunscreen, the zinc oxide, and the oils. You can follow the exact measurements that I have suggested for the oils, or you can add or take away as many drops as you like.

You are going to get incredible benefits from all the oils regardless of how much you use, but you will get more benefits depending on how much you use.

Use your blender until the mix is light and whipped, then transfer to a glass jar.

Store with the lid screwed on tightly, and massage into your skin when you are ready to use.

The Cali Keys

13 drops jasmine

7 drops Melissa

5 drops sandalwood

Base

Directions:

In a mixing bowl, blend all of the ingredients, first the base for the sunscreen, the zinc oxide, and the oils. You can follow the exact measurements that I have suggested for the oils, or you can add or take away as many drops as you like.

You are going to get incredible benefits from all the oils regardless of how much you use, but you will get more benefits depending on how much you use.

Use your blender until the mix is light and whipped, then transfer to a glass jar.

Store with the lid screwed on tightly, and massage into your skin when you are ready to use.

The Carefreedom Ring Blend

8 drops neroli

4 drops parsley

5 drops chamomile

4 drops myrrh

5 drops jasmine

Base

Directions:

In a mixing bowl, blend all of the ingredients, first the base for the sunscreen, the zinc oxide, and the oils. You can follow the exact measurements that I have suggested for the oils, or you can add or take away as many drops as you like.

You are going to get incredible benefits from all the oils regardless of how much you use, but you will get more benefits depending on how much you use.

Use your blender until the mix is light and whipped, then transfer to a glass jar.

Store with the lid screwed on tightly, and massage into your skin when you are ready to use.

Conclusion

There you have it, everything you need to know to make your own sunscreen, and to make it be everything you want it to be, and then some. If you have ever studied the use of essential oils, you know that there are all kinds of health benefits that come from using it.

There are more than one benefit that comes from making your own lotion. To name a few, you are going to be able to avoid all of the harmful chemicals that are placed into normal lotions, you will be able to choose your own scents, your own style, and your own flavors.

You will be able to choose lotions that have other benefits in addition to the protection from the sun, including cutting down on the acne, cutting down on your wrinkles, and even smoothing rough skin. You are going to see your blemishes vanish, and gain even more protection from the sun.

There's no end to the ways you can make these your own, and I hope this book was able to show you how. There's no need to stress, no need to give up and go with the different kinds of lotions they have on the shelves in the store, and no need to give up and spend an arm and a leg to get the good kind of lotion.

I hope this book was able to show you that you can have it all, and you can have it your way. You don't need to settle for something that isn't your preferred flavor. You don't need to settle for something that you don't like, and you don't need to spend money on something that is more than you need.

You have been out in the sun so many times, you know that a simple sunscreen doesn't cut it. You have to get what you are after, or you are going to get left in the sun, and your skin is going to show the negative results.

With this book, you are going to learn how to make any and all kinds of sunscreen, and you are going to see the wonderful results that come from using it. No burns, no peeling skin, and no hassle. This is truly your best friend when it comes to sunscreen, and you won't ever want to go back to the other options any more.

So don't wait another day, you can get anything you want, exactly as you want it. Go ahead, jump in with both feet!

www.ingramcontent.com/pod-product-compliance
Lightning Source LLC
Chambersburg PA
CBHW061934280526
45787CB00004B/1595